Lucien A.E. Manga

Climate change, health and

development in Africa

What policy-makers need to understand

Acknowledgments

This booklet contains the perceptions and views of the author only and does not represent the decisions or stated policies of the World Health Organization.

I owe special gratitude to Dicky Akanmori for his help with technical review and to Kellen Kebaara for language editing.

My sincere thanks also go to Bernadette Ramirez, Pierre Quiblier and Xavier Daney for their advice.

Contents

Foreword

This booklet has been written for all those interested in understanding climate change and its relationship with public health and development in Africa. It is meant primarily to help policy- and decision-makers but also the wider audience to appreciate that climate change should now be part of every policy and programmatic decision. It also provides arguments for a paradigm shift and encourages African leaders to see in climate change an excellent opportunity for development. The booklet is intended as a contribution to the knowledge base for development in Africa.

Acronyms and abbreviations

AR5	Fifth assessment report
ARVs	Antiretroviral
CDM	Clean Development Mechanism
GFCS	Global Framework for Climate Services
HIV/AIDS	Human immunodeficiency virus/ infection/ acquired immune deficiency syndrome
IPCC	Intergovernmental Panel on Climate Change
NAPA	National adaptation programmes of action
UN-REDD	Reducing Emissions from Deforestation and forest Degradation in developing countries
SPM	Summary For Policy Makers
UNFCCC	United Nations Framework Convention on Climate Change
USEPA	United States Environmental Protection Agency
WHO	World Health Organization

Introduction

Even after more than 60 years of political independence, Africa is still a continent characterized by underdevelopment, poverty and disease. Indeed, 34 out of the 48 countries classified as the least developed by the United Nations are in Africa.[1] The poverty rate, which is the head count ratio at US\$ 1.25 a day, was 46.8% in 2011.[2] In spite of the modest progress witnessed in the recent past, the overall burden of disease is highest on the African continent.[3]

The recent past has seen an indication of consistent economic growth over a few years as assessed on the basis of the annual gross domestic product (GDP). On average, the estimated annual growth in GDP was 4.1% in 2013. The prospects indicate that this will be sustained over the next several years. The current economic patterns, if maintained, will certainly translate into prosperity for the continent.

Healthy people are an asset for a country's development. A nation cannot develop harmoniously without healthy people. In Africa, regretfully, national investments in health are still largely inadequate, as they constitute less than 15% of the national budget in most countries. In spite of this, there have been some gains in public health in the continent over the recent past. The reductions in HIV/AIDS transmission and in malaria mortality, as well as the improvements in child mortality indicators, are some of the examples. Unfortunately, natural disasters, and particularly climate change, threaten to erode many of these gains.

Climate change is, as emphasized by the *Lancet*, "the biggest global health threat of the 21st century".[4] Its adverse impacts on health and development are increasingly being recognized and are important. Broad national policies, strategies and plans for climate change mitigation and adaptation already exist. National platforms have been established to coordinate implementation of these policies in African countries. Climate change adaptation could be turned into a development opportunity for Africa but action is still lacking.

Climate change adaptation, especially in the health sector, provides an exceptional opportunity for governments to accelerate their country's economic and social development by investing in it a part of the additional income generated from economic growth. This booklet aims to provide some perspectives to that end to national policy-makers.

What is climate change?

There have been and there will continue to be debate and controversy over whether climate change is a myth or a reality. Whatever the answer is to that question, the fact is that climatic factors have adverse effects and impacts on the health and well-being of individuals. The exact definition of climate change itself is a matter of debate and is dependent on the background of those giving it.

According to the Intergovernmental Panel on Climate Change (IPCC), climate change refers to a change in the state of the climate that can be identified, using statistical tests for example, by changes in the mean and/or the variability of its properties and that persists for an extended period, typically decades or longer. It is any change in climate over time, whether it is due to natural variability or it is as a result of human activity.[5]

For the United Nations Framework Convention on Climate Change (UNFCCC), climate change means a change in climate that is attributed directly or indirectly to human activity, that alters the composition of the global atmosphere and that, in addition to the natural climate variability, is observed over comparable time periods.[6]

The United States Environmental Protection Agency (USEPA) defines climate change as any significant change in the measures of climate lasting for an extended period of time. In other words, climate change includes major changes in temperature, precipitation or wind patterns that occur over several decades or longer.[7]

These definitions carry the nuances associated with the differences in the perspectives of the bodies from which they originate. For IPCC, the emphasis is on the rigorous and scientific demonstration that climate features are unstable and have coherent trends over time, irrespective of what determines such instability. IPCC members are scientists. They work to generate scientific knowledge. What is essential for them is the unquestionable evidence that they must generate.

For UNFCCC, the critical issue to be addressed relates to the proportion of change that could be directly or indirectly attributable to human activity, or what is termed anthropogenic climate change. The basis of this lies within the mandate of UNFCCC, which is to ensure that anthropogenic climate change is halted and reversed through the reduction of the greenhouse gases resulting from human activity.

To USEPA, which is a national regulatory body, what matters is that the public understand in simple terms what climate change could mean and that the afferent national policies, legislation and guidelines can be implemented effectively by everyone.

The Fifth Assessment Report (AR5) of IPCC indicates that the globally averaged combined land and ocean temperature data as calculated by a linear trend show a warming of 0.85 °C over the period 1880–2012, for which multiple, independently produced data sets exist, and about 0.89 °C for 1901–2012 and 0.72 °C for 1951–2012, based on three independently produced data sets. The total increase between the averages for the 1850–1900 and 2003–2012 periods is 0.78 °C.[8] The same report notes, on the other hand, that "Despite the robust multi-decadal warming, there exists substantial inter-annual to decadal variability in the rate of warming, with several periods exhibiting weaker trends". The increasing trend in temperature of the earth's surface over the past century, coupled with the notable temperature variability over shorter periods, needs to be noted.

What does this knowledge mean for public health? Public health professionals must agree on a common understanding of climate change. It is not that they require their own definition of the phenomenon but that they interpret the climate change definition in the same way. It is generally understood that climatic factors are essential health determinants. For example, malaria transmission patterns are associated with seasons.

Generally, and even though this is not always correct, the rainy season is associated with high malaria transmission, while the dry season corresponds with the low malaria transmission period. Rainfall patterns, therefore, are the critical determinant of malaria epidemiology. This is known and well understood by the communities that malaria affects as well as public health professionals. What is less clear is that, now with climate change, there is increased variability in these factors with significant public health and development consequences. Rainfall could be significantly higher than usual during the dry season in certain areas where usually only a few malaria cases are expected. This would result in malaria epidemics with high case fatality rates, because the appropriate epidemic response would be delayed. The delay itself would be due to a lack of epidemic preparedness.

Unexpected variations in temperature may lead to a significant increase in conditions associated with heat stress in areas where such conditions are not normally witnessed. Medical teams need to relate such phenomena to climate change so that they can factor these trends in planning and capacity development for heat stress management. Because the variability of climate results in changes in the epidemiological patterns of disease, the common understanding that public health professionals should have is that the unexpected changes that are currently being observed in climate-sensitive diseases have to be considered as the effects of climate change and addressed in that context. For public health professionals and decision-makers that is what counts the most in the matter of climate change.

Lessons from recent IPCC assessments and their implications for public health

The key messages from IPCC's 5th Synthesis Report (2014), which are contained in the 'Summary for policy makers', have to be analysed and interpreted from the public health perspective. These messages provide a solid basis for immediate action by governments. While most, if not all, of the messages have health implications, some of them are of more direct value to health policies than are others.

IPCC's key messages

SPM 1. Observed changes and their causes: Human influence on the climate system is clear, and recent anthropogenic emissions of greenhouse gases are the highest in history. Recent climate changes have had widespread impacts on human and natural systems.

SPM 2. Future climate changes, risks and impacts: Continued emission of greenhouse gases will cause further warming and long-lasting changes in all components of the climate system, increasing the likelihood of severe, pervasive and irreversible impacts for people and ecosystems. Limiting climate change would require substantial and sustained reductions in greenhouse gas emissions which, together with adaptation, can limit climate change risks.

SPM 3. Future pathways for adaptation, mitigation and sustainable development: Adaptation and mitigation are complementary strategies for reducing and managing the risks of climate change. Substantial emissions reductions over the next few decades can reduce climate risks in the 21st century and beyond, increase prospects for effective adaptation, reduce the costs and challenges of mitigation in the longer term, and contribute to climate-resilient pathways for sustainable development.

SPM 4. Adaptation and mitigation: Many adaptation and mitigation options can help address climate change, but no single option is sufficient by itself. Effective implementation depends on policies and cooperation at all scales, and can be enhanced through integrated responses that link adaptation and mitigation with other societal objectives.

Programming of public health actions needs to shift from an approach based on a predictable disease burden and fixed budgets to control them to one based on an unpredictable disease burden and contingency health budgets. Today, most public health planners use historical data and trends to define interventions and to determine the levels of resources required. This now has to gradually change. The new public health planning paradigm should accommodate measures to manage uncertainties. More importantly, it should use information generated from environmental surveillance and climate forecasting. This is true not for only health but for all development sectors.

The variability observed in climate change that is detrimental to public health will continue to occur and will even exacerbate. One could assume that there may be a one-off epidemiological transition for climate-sensitive diseases and expect stability at a point in time. That is very unlikely. What IPCC affirms is that the variability in climate factors will continue to occur and to intensify for decades, which means that the epidemiology of most climate-sensitive diseases and health conditions will be more and more difficult to understand or address with the tools available today. Therefore, steps should be taken now for public health preparedness in anticipation of even more changes in the future.

The sound management of climate change impacts on public health will depend to a large extent on the availability of good tools and models for prediction and forecasting. To fill the current research gap in the development and application of such tools, strong collaboration is required between African scientists and institutions and those from other parts of the world. Public health experts need to learn from the long history of collaboration between sectors such as agriculture and the water with hydro-meteorological services. The Famine Early Warning Systems Network (FEWS NET) is an example worth emulating. FEWS NET has succeeded in using metrological information to establish effective early warning systems for prediction and sound management of food insecurity in many parts of the world.[9]

The use of climate information for development is so important that the World Meteorological Organization, a specialized agency of the United Nations, has established a Global Framework for Climate Services (GFCS) with the vision to "enable better management of the risks of climate variability and change and adaptation to climate change, through the development and incorporation of science-based climate information and prediction into planning, policy and practice on the global, regional and national scale".[10] One of the focal areas of GFCS is health. GFCS intends to bring hydro-meteorological services to work more closely with epidemiologists and public health planners to improve disease forecasting. This work is starting now, though timidly, mostly from the research side.

Some scientists in Africa have been able to use climate information to develop predictive models for disease epidemics. Such work needs to be scaled up. It is expected that partnerships such as the International Consortium for Climate and Health in Africa (Clim-HEALTH Africa), which is a global collaboration of leading institutions in the area of climate change and health, which is coordinated by WHO and which builds up from previous similar initiatives will play a key role in that context.[11]

Public health systems so far have been ineffective in disease prevention in general and disease risk management in particular. Often, health information systems are built to generate information on current situations and trends, but even this they do mostly in an unsatisfactory manner. Disease risk identification, mapping and management are some of the weakest areas in disease prevention and control in Africa. This is linked to the very low priority accorded to preventive services in comparison with curative services. We are learning that climate change will amplify existing risks and create new ones for natural and human-made systems. What specific risks? when? where? and how? are essential questions that national public health authorities must start to answer.

Most ministries of health do not yet have specific units dealing with the health effects of climate change. Many countries are setting up working groups on climate and health that bring together mostly meteorological staff and health experts to discuss climate change and health issues. But a number of these groups are still informal and do not have decision-making powers nor resources do carry out their work. It is now indispensable to establish specific climate change and health units within the ministries of health to not only find answers to the questions above but also provide comprehensive leadership for the broad scope of work that needs to be undertaken now to more systematically address the health impacts of climate change.

Most African governments tend to react rather than be proactive. In public health terms, surveillance systems, especially for infectious diseases, are not conceptualized and built to meet the requirements of climate change adaptation. In other words, surveillance needs to shift from a case-based model to risk monitoring. Analytical frameworks and modelling for sensitive climate and disease predictions for the short and medium terms are starting to emerge, but they are still limited to research purposes. The close collaboration required among the ministries of health, the ministries of environment, and hydro-meteorological services, as provided for in the Libreville Declaration on Health and Environment in Africa, is yet to materialize.

The IPCC messages highlight the fact that more than ever before, governments must ensure cohesion of the policies of the various development sectors to be able to bring together climate change mitigation and adaptation pathways, rather than keeping them separate as is the case today. Public health policies themselves must be revamped to accommodate climate change mitigation and adaptation measures. An approach such as 'greening the health sector' that has been initiated by some United Nations agencies can have a catalytic impact on the sectors dealing with climate change adaptation.

Public health impacts of climate change

Strictly speaking, the health impacts of climate change refer to the incremental disease burden that can be attributed to the change in the climate at a specific location. Those impacts are assessed based on the correlation, whether positive or negative, of a specific disease trend with trends in the anomalies of one or multiple climatic factors in the same location over a multi-decadal time frame.

As surprising as it might seem, there is scarce evidence so far on the impacts of climate change as such on public health. Only a few studies have been able to directly incriminate climate change for the increase in the burden of specific diseases or health conditions and to quantify such increases. The reasons are related but not limited to the definition of climate change, the data requirements and the many probable confounding factors.

One of the few studies that have demonstrated the impact of climate change on public health was undertaken in the highlands of Kenya. Alonso and colleagues[12] analysed the trends in monthly mean temperatures from records from two meteorological stations within tea estates in the highlands of Kenya and had them correlated with confirmed malaria cases from records of inpatients from those tea estates over the period 1970–2002. They demonstrated a positive correlation between the rise in the mean temperature and the increase in malaria cases.[12]

From the definition of climate change, an analysis of the trend in climate anomalies over multiple decades (usually 30 years or so) is required before climate change could be considered responsible for any impact on health. Variations in climatic factors over shorter periods than that, even if they are positively correlated with observed increases in certain diseases, will not qualify as emanating from climate change impact. They will be simply associated with climate variability.

If you search the PubMed literature database using 'climate change, public health impacts, Africa' as key words, you will be very surprised that most of the publications pulled up that will refer to public health impacts of climate change in their titles will actually be on public health impacts of climate variability. Increased climate variability is one of the main characteristics of climate change, but climate variability alone is not climate change.

For researchers to incriminate climate change as the driver of epidemiological changes in any given location, they must rely on two important data sets: consistent measurements of climatic parameters (essentially temperature and rainfall) over 3 decades at least and consistent measurements of specific diseases or health conditions in the same location over the same period. Unfortunately, finding suitable locations with such data sets in Africa is difficult. This is due to the fact that historically, the development and coverage of hydro-meteorological services have been inadequate and uneven in most African countries. Even when such data exist, access to them remains very limited and difficult, mainly because the associated administrative processes are ineffective and that in many instances researchers need to pay for such information. On the part of public health, national health information systems remain mostly in their embryological stage. They do not always have readily available and usable health information. In addition, when data that exist are cleaned, those of poor quality might be discarded in the process.

Development processes themselves are likely to be responsible for a great deal of the changes in certain locations that are similar to those generated by climate variability. Urbanization, environmental degradation, demographical factors and development projects represent weighty confounding factors in statistical analysis in view of the requirement for long time series data. Obviously, direct observation of climate change impacts on public health has difficult challenges. Byass's 2009 review[13] of this issue provides an interesting perspective. The situation has not changed much since then.

The challenges in categorizing the impact of climate change on health have led scientists to choose to develop and use mathematical models to estimate the burden of disease attributable to the impact of climate change on human health. Raw WHO estimates indicated that of the worldwide deaths in 2004, climate change was responsible for 3% of those from diarrhoea, 3%

of those from malaria and 3.8% of those from dengue fever. The total mortality attributable to climate change in 2004 was about 0.2%, of which 85% was among children.[14]

Climate change affects health and well-being in several ways, but mainly it is through the direct or indirect exposure of humans to unusual levels of climate parameters using environmental, social and economic pathways. The Atlas of Health and Climate published by WHO in 2012[15] lists and categorizes diseases and public health conditions that are sensitive to climate and, therefore, climate change. It also describes some of the documented impacts of climatic factors on health, as well as defining the future changes that might occur in the epidemiology of certain diseases as a result of climate change. The Atlas serves as an important source of information to identify specific diseases and conditions and to map the areas that may be more likely than others to be affected by climate change.

Malaria, one of the most studied vector-borne diseases, is also one of the best diseases to use in examples to illustrate how climate change directly or indirectly affects health. Temperature, rainfall and humidity are the climate factors that influence the breeding and survival rates of the *Anopheles* mosquito, the malaria vector. Changes in any of these parameters have immediate impact on the vector levels, abundance, survival rates and eventual vectorial capacity, that is the capacity to transmit the parasite. One important element is the fact that the development of the malaria parasite within the mosquito itself is also affected by temperature. If the temperature is lower than 18 °C, the part of the biological cycle of the malaria parasite that takes place within the mosquito will be aborted and the mosquito will not be capable of transmitting malaria. This is why normally malaria transmission does not occur in highlands beyond about 1700 m above sea level. Some of the worst malaria epidemics that have occurred in the highlands of Ethiopia and Madagascar among others are attributed to changes in temperature in those areas, an aspect of climate variability. There have also been reports of increases in malaria cases in the higher altitudes of Burundi and Rwanda, where malaria was not seen in the past.

Climate factors are important determinants of all vector-borne diseases and others that are transmitted by intermediary hosts. These include dengue, yellow fever, trypanosomiasis, onchorcerciasis, lymphatic filariasis, schistosomiais etc. The specific epidemiology of these diseases will be affected through the life cycles of their vectors, but not necessarily in the same way. In some situations the impacts could be the opposite of what is expected. For instance, it might happen that the scarcity of rain results in severe drought, which, in turn, reduces malaria transmission. But the fact that households would have to store water provisions at home and often in uncovered containers would favour the increase of *Aedes* mosquitoes with the potential for bringing on outbreaks of arbovirus diseases such as yellow fever or chikungunya. This is because, unlike *Anopheles* mosquitoes, which breed in water pools usually created by rain, *Aedes* mosquitoes breed in water containers usually in the home surroundings.

Since the relationships between the variation in climatic factors and disease outcomes may not always be as expected, only frequent monitoring of the determinants by public health experts and health risks assessments can provide the necessary information to guide planning, resource allocation and operations. This is the reason that an integrated environment and health surveillance approach is of utmost importance.

The example given about the impacts of climatic factors on the variability in the epidemiology of vector-borne diseases is meant to only exemplify how climate risks interfere with human health. Almost every other disease or health condition will be affected by climate variability and change. Waterborne diseases, for instance, are very susceptible to climate change. Rainfall patterns are an important determinant of the epidemiology of waterborne diseases. The frequency of cholera outbreaks in the parts of Africa with low coverage of water and sanitation facilities can be associated with rainfall variability. Similarly, food availability and, therefore, the nutritional status of communities, which are intrinsically linked with crop production, are associated with rainfall patterns as well. In addition, the increased need for communities to conserve food as security measure against famine during droughts but in inadequate storage facilities exposes them to the risk of outbreaks of food-borne diseases.

Beyond temperature and rainfall, climatic factors such as wind and dust are proven to be key determinants of infectious disease epidemiology, as is the case with meningitis. The Atlas of Climate and Health of WHO[15] alludes to the fact that there is a clear seasonal pattern of meningitis cases that corresponds to the period of the year when there are increases in dust concentrations and reductions in the intertropical convergence zone winds.

Climate change affects noncommunicable diseases also such as heat stress and mental health. Heat stress is known to have caused hundreds of deaths in Europe in recent years. This could also be the case in some parts of Africa. Research is going on in southern Africa to relate climate change to increases in heath stress. A significant increase in asthma was observed in the United States between 2001 and 2011.[16]

Impact of climate change on health systems

Building and maintaining a health facility are significant investments for a government or any other health provider. The loss of or damage to such a unit would have important implications for the beneficiaries, for it would deprive them of basic health services for a long period, because reconstruction would not be undertaken or completed immediately. Access to health services would be minimal in the meantime, with potential increases in morbidity and mortality and worsening of health indicators.

Governments develop their national health strategic plans and budgets based on assumptions regarding the burden of disease that they have to address. The information used to define the magnitude of the disease burden itself is generally based on estimates. Often, in the course of the implementation of the strategic plan the disease burden will change unexpectedly but significantly because of extreme weather events. Without adequate emergency preparedness, which is often the case, many of these events evolve into disasters.

The most visible impacts of climate change on public health are those that are direct and immediate. These are either the impacts of extreme weather events or climate-induced disasters. Some of these impacts can be anticipated if weather predictions are made available in sufficient time.

In normal circumstances, the health care system is organized in a way to provide some basic services at the very local level, such as management of malaria cases or of childhood illness. Either community health workers or household members themselves do this. A number of community health programmes have advanced to a level where, for instance, village vendors have turned into pharmacists with a certain degree of success, at least at the experimental stage. Health commodities including drugs such as antimalarials or disease-preventive commodities such as mosquito nets or condoms could be accessed through such local vendors.

Floods destroy first and foremost shelters and what they contain. In the event of mild floods with low or no displacement of populations, stocks of medicines or preventive commodities might be damaged and years of efforts ruined. Community members in many cases contribute to the financing of health services at the local level. It should be noted that mild flooding incidents are frequent and are underreported, so it can be anticipated that when the loss and damage from such events are summed up the levels will be unexpectedly high.

Severe floods have much greater direct impact than mild flooding. They not only affect much wider areas but also because of their intensity they cause massive population displacement, often of about a hundred thousand people. In these situations, the priority of individuals and their families is simply to survive, as these events are always associated with drowning and death. In addition, they interrupt community level health services, meaning that providing assistance to those affected by illness or death will not be possible. Counselling, case management, safe delivery and other services will stop.

Community health services represent a substantial and growing component of health care delivery systems in Africa. Unfortunately, most of the time they are left out of the essential actions for disaster response, relief and reconstruction services. Although the tools applied to quantify and map health services availability after disaster accord attention to community health services and health facilities, the recovery and reconstruction programmes which are be based on information provided by these assessments often have minimal consideration of the community health component. Policy-makers and professionals in disaster and risk management must redress these gaps.

The deterioration in environmental conditions in the areas affected by flooding results in increases in the levels of malaria, diarrhoeal diseases, acute respiratory infections, malnutrition etc., which are the leading causes of morbidity and mortality in such cases. Mobile clinics are one of the solutions proposed to ensure that basic services are provided during such disasters, but because of flooding and destruction of the road infrastructure, such clinics will be restricted to only accessible areas.

The management of chronic diseases and conditions such as diabetes, hypertension, HIV/AIDS and cancer is not prioritized in the essential health services offered to communities during flooding, because the focus is mostly on communicable diseases. Emergency obstetrical and neonatal care are likely to disappear. This is complicated by the fact that many health workers who live and work in the affected areas will themselves be victims of the disaster and will be concerned only about their personal survival and that of their family.

The destruction of the road infrastructure and telecommunications equipment will have far-reaching and direct impact on health systems' components. The management of referral services for health conditions such as severe injuries, pregnancies requiring emergency obstetrical care, severe malaria etc. will be a challenge. Fatalities related to these conditions will increase. Medical supply stockpiles will be lost, but their replenishment will be difficult because the supply chains will not be able to function. Cold chains, which are indispensable for immunization services, as well as the logistic functions for other preventive services such as distribution of bednets or condoms will not be able work either. The net result of all these failures in the health system will be a reduction in the coverage of health interventions, followed by an increase in the incidence of the respective diseases. Epidemics of measles, malaria and cholera are markers of the failure of the health system in emergency situations.

Health information systems are not yet fully computerized in most parts of Africa and patient records are still paper based. Peripheral health facilities collect and collate data on registers and compile information on sheets and then send these to the next level, which is always the districts, where a first compilation of data and analysis are done. This stage does not include data cleaning. The shortcomings in this process are known and they include flawed and inconsistent data, gaps in information etc. When health information systems' managers need to conduct systematic and scientific analyses of the health situation and trends (this is even more important for research on epidemiology), they have to go back to the primary source of information, which is the health facilities' records. The loss of registers and files in flooded health facilities creates an unbridgeable gap in historical data from the affected area. When this affects other important services that collect information that could serve the purpose of public health at the local level such as meteorological or administrative services, the consequences are even dire.

Droughts also have specific impacts on health systems, although such impacts are less spectacular or evident than those associated with flooding. It is well known that infection prevention and control measures, including hygiene techniques, are weakly applied in most African settings and, in particular, in the rural areas, where access to water and sanitation facilities is inadequate. Water scarcity that comes with drought worsens the implementation of infection prevention measures. This by itself may increase the risk of nosocomial infections. On the other hand, the increase in diseases such as meningitis and trachoma and conditions such as acute malnutrition in children is likely to overwhelm the health facilities. The rise in the risk of fires also may directly or indirectly affect the health systems through increasing casualties and fatalities.

There are other less visible but equally or more important impacts. Those impacts are indirect, of medium or long term nature and related to the slowdown in the implementation of public health programmes, worsening of health indicators and loss of public health gains.

African governments need to understand and respond to climate variability and uncertainty. The management of disaster risk-reduction programmes in many parts of the world provides ample examples on efficient and effective approaches to anticipate and respond to disastrous environmental risks. Unfortunately, the implementation of disaster risk-reduction frameworks such and the Hyogo Framework for Action, which came into force in 2005 and will conclude in 2015, has been mediocre in general. This is in spite of the increasing occurrence of natural disasters in Africa, including extreme weather events due to climate change.

Adaptation to climate change in the health sector

A study published in 2013 on health considerations within national adaptation programmes of action (NAPAs) in developing countries and small island developing states[17] concluded that, with only a few exceptions, the consideration of public health interventions in NAPAs needed to be strengthened to support the resiliency processes and protect public health from the negative effects of climate change. It recommended that the ministries of health establish specific task teams to undertake the required work relating to vulnerability assessments and adaptation planning.

Vulnerability assessments and adaptation planning can be daunting tasks. Vulnerability assessments are undertaken to basically understand the extent to which climate anomalies will affect public health and health systems.

Adaptation planning aims to ensure that clear objectives are set to mitigate the effects of climate impacts on public health and health systems, and ensure that actions are defined and resources set aside to that end.

To date, few African country are known to have set up the teams for vulnerability assessment or adaptation planning and have undertaken the needed preparatory work. The reasons for this are many. In spite of all the extreme events reported on the continent and their adverse effects on public health and development, the impacts of climate change have not yet swayed the consciousness of public health policy-makers to the extent that they feel impelled to change priorities and catalyse and accelerate climate change adaptation actions. But even if they had done so, national and international expertise, as well as financial resources, are still largely inadequate to meet the needs of African countries. Insufficient domestic resources as well as limited international technical and financial assistance characterize the current context.

Technical resources for climate change adaptation such as guidelines, assessment tools and specific information management systems are still insufficient. It must be remembered that since their independence, African countries have been struggling even with trying to attain their national health objectives. This is due in part to the enormous challenges they confront in developing satisfactory health systems. Climate change is a new and major challenge adding on to those already in existence.

But despite the challenges, one must have a vision of an African continent that is effectively and efficiently adapting to climate change. In reality, the effects of climate change have been identified and felt by many local communities for decades. Agricultural communities, for example, have noted inconsistencies and variations in seasons as they relate to sowing periods. It is possible that some of these communities have had to change their practices and have become more resilient to the changes. That is what adaptation essentially is. The extent to which African communities have empirically perceived climate change and adapted to it deserves more investigation. There will be many lessons to be learnt from that.

Interestingly, the health sector is one of the few for which a clear way forward for climate change adaptation has been defined at the continental level. Strategic and programmatic actions have been identified in the context of the WHO Pan African Programme for Public Health Adaptation to Climate Change. The resources required also have been estimated for the medium term. This is the result of a policy dialogue between the ministers of health and the ministers of the environment, which led to the development of the 'Framework for Public Health Adaptation to

Climate Change'. A five-year action plan for the continent was subsequently developed by WHO[18] with five objectives: (1) identification of country-specific health risks associated with climate change, (2) strengthening of core national capacities that enable health systems to prepare for and effectively respond to climate change threats to human health, (3) facilitation of the implementation of integrated essential public health and environment interventions, (4) operational and applied research on local health adaptation needs and solutions, and (5) dissemination of lessons learnt and country experiences.

Up to now, all the African countries have been able to do is prepare their specific health adaptation plans. A few of them have also started to receive catalytic funds to initiate some demonstration projects from their development partners. This is a good step forward but is largely insufficient.

A question that should be raised is whether governments should have specific adaptation programmes at the sector level. This is an important governance issue for them. Doing so would require that each sector has its own national adaptation programme, which would mean that health, agriculture, water resources etc. would have to compete for priority consideration and resources. Operating the programmes would require enormous coordination efforts. But this seems to be the current trend. Although UNFCCC has so far succeeded to minimize sector-specific discussions in climate change negotiations, pressure from activists from various sectors is starting to change this situation.

It might be wiser for governments to establish technical institutions for climate change to address the specific needs of the various sectors but to integrate adaptation programmes and projects as much as possible. In the case of health, the adaptation programmes would need to focus on building resilient health care systems. For the curative services, this requires health facilities that will withstand floods and droughts, alternative referral systems to be activated during extreme weather events and special arrangements and facilities to protect health care workers, including those in the communities. The preventive services will need to focus on intensification of the disease prevention programmes such as immunization.

Immunization is the greatest short-term climate change adaptation intervention that exists today. If all children could be fully immunized on time, there would be an immediate reduction in vulnerabilities to all vaccine-preventable diseases such as measles, polio, tetanus, meningitis and yellow fever, which would be one of the greatest progresses in the adaptation of public health to climate change. Other preventive interventions such as the wide use of bednets with sufficient coverage are possible, but they pose much bigger challenges related to their cost, the need to be frequently replaced and, more importantly, adherence to their systematic use.

Reorienting national policies to accelerate effective adaptation to climate change

The character of the policy reforms that are required to meaningfully address climate change is such that they can only and effectively be addressed if they become embedded in national laws. African governments must therefore seriously consider including minimum requirements for climate change adaptation in their national legislative and human rights frameworks. A national policy dialogue drawing input from all stakeholders could be an effective means of achieving this. An important incentive will be the many development opportunities that will arise from climate change adaptation activities.

Adapting to climate change in the health sector requires a shift from the 'business as usual' mode of thinking and operating to more audacious approaches. African governments must appreciate the value of and develop and implement policies that favour risk management approaches.

Lessons on disaster risk management from the experiences of Turkey and Mexico, among others, must be leant and applied. Following major disasters that resulted from earthquakes and hurricanes, these two countries adopted stringent public policies that have made their communities resilient to such calamities. What those policies have in common is the optimal accommodation of social dimensions. Their implementation relies not only on legislation but also on dialogue with beneficiary communities, coupled with sound financial mechanisms, clear guidelines and accountability frameworks.[19] In Turkey, "by the Act dated 29/5/2009 and No. 5902 Establishment of Disaster and Emergency Management Presidency; General Directorate of

Turkey Emergency Management under Prime Ministry, General Directorate of Civil Defence under Ministry of Interior, General Directorate of Disaster Affairs under Ministry of Public Works and Settlement were closed. Three core institutions have unified under a single independent authority with the act adopted by the Parliament and entered into force in June 2009".

The policy and institutional transformation came after this country had suffered two consecutive and devastating earthquakes in 1999. These prompted the national authorities to work with academia and other stakeholders and to adopt a major shift of approach to policy formulation and implementation from disaster response to risk assessment and management.

In Mexico, the cumulative cost of the disasters between 2000 and 2010 is estimated to have totalled more than US$ 25.1 billion. The three events with the greatest magnitude of damage were the 1985 earthquake, Hurricane Wilma of

2005 and Hurricane Alex of 2010.[20] It is the Mexico City earthquake of 1985 that served as the catalyst for a new approach to disaster risk management in the country. That earthquake caused a loss estimated at about US$ 12 billion. Mexico now practises multidisciplinary approaches involving all stakeholders for effective risk assessment and mitigation, working through the National System of Civil Protection, a unified institution established in 1986. The country has been so successful with its disaster risk management programme that it has been recognized with strong backing from the World Bank, which recently supported a US$ 315 million catastrophe bond providing insurance against earthquakes and hurricanes.[21]

African countries can easily adopt the Turkish or Mexican policy philosophy and processes for disaster risk management in general and climate change adaptation in particular. It is the duty of national policy-makers to understand the needs and opportunities relating to climate change and to take the necessary pertinent actions.

African countries have signed the Hyogo Framework for Action on disaster risk management and they have established national platforms to coordinate the actions of the relevant sectors to respond to disasters. Also, the health sector is represented in these national coordination mechanisms. But health concerns are not being moved to the forefront of national contingency plans. For example, very few countries have established functioning national emergency funds to respond to emergencies and disasters including those created by climate change. Therefore, when such events occur, identification and allocation of the funding required for response can be lengthy processes, and usually the funds are taken from existing programmes. This, of course, means that many of the activities of these regular programmes will become underfunded and insufficiently implemented, and their objectives will not be realized. In addition, the rehabilitation and recovery phases that follow acute response in emergency management may prioritize reconstruction of infrastructure and absorb the limited available resources, even though a good share of these are provided by the international assistance community for emergency and disaster response.

The Third United Nations World Conference on Disaster Risk Reduction, which took place in Sendai, Japan, on 14 to 18 March 2015, demonstrated that disaster risk reduction is progressively being steadfastly integrated as an essential component of national policies and plans in many parts of the world. Climate change adaptation is articulated well as an element in disaster mitigation in the Sendai Framework for Disaster Risk Reduction, as is health. This action-oriented framework provides an important opportunity for the health sector to address climate change more comprehensively and effectively.

For the health sector to execute the role it was assigned by the Sendai Framework for Disaster Risk Reduction, the ministries of health will need to be more proactive and engaged in national disaster risk reduction platforms. Some of their key actions would be the creation and resourcing of national multidisciplinary public health risk-management teams with climate change adaptation as one of their assigned mandates. Their responsibilities will be to develop and implement national early warning systems based on both iterative risk assessments and disease surveillance. Enough national experts should be trained for that purpose. The teams should also undertake research on trends in climate change risks and their potential impacts on health. Africa currently does not have enough scientists who understand climate change and its impacts of on health. This research must be linked to national capacity development in the health sector and the use of meteorological information to plan for adaptation programmes. The Global Framework for Climate Services offers many illustrations in those areas.

The development of multisectoral programmes that link health, environment, land and other sectors can help to map and manage flood-prone areas. National standards for construction need to be developed, even for rural settings. Relocation areas, or safe heavens, need to be identified and prepared for the quick accommodation of displaced populations in the event of floods. The relevant recommendations from the Health Safety Index initiative, which helps governments to build resilient health facilities, should be implemented in Africa as a matter of urgency.

There should be a health approach to climate change. An important area of work in national policies and institutional arrangements is the setting up of public health units in all government departments. Such an arrangement would speed up the implementation process for the health component in all policies, an approach that is now being promoted by WHO, but will also facilitate dialogue between the health sector and the other sectors. One of the main roles of the health units in these departments will be to ensure that policies, strategies, programmes and projects comply with public health requirements and contain measures that promote climate change adaptation.

Climate change and equity, human rights, governance and health

There are fundamental issues that need to be addressed regarding equity, human rights, governance and health as they relate to climate change. In Africa, access to health and health care is characterized by wide inequities. Mutangadura and colleagues[22] document large inequities in accessing health care that are due to income differences and location. They demonstrate that specific policies aimed at improving both geographical and financial access to health care are essential and that scaling up of pro-poor strategies and increased health service provision in underserved areas are crucial.

It can be anticipated that climate change will worsen the inequities and disparities in access to health care. Why? Because wealthier people will tend to move from the areas that are prone to climate-related disasters to settle in the less vulnerable zones. Or they will have the resources to build living environments that will be more resilient to climate impacts. In either case, their access to health care services will be significantly better compared to that of the poor people. Climate change will exacerbate health inequalities and disparities and will have as the ultimate consequence much higher morbidity and mortality rates in the poorer communities.

There is an urgent need to implement and scale up pro-poor public health policies such as universal health coverage,[1] but perhaps what is even more pressing is the need to embrace the right-to-health approaches and to pre-eminently enforce them. There are key questions to be

[1] WHO defines universal health coverage as ensuring that all people can use the promotive, preventive, curative, rehabilitative and palliative health services they need, of sufficient quality to be effective, while also ensuring that the use of these services does not expose the user to financial hardship.

answered in this context: Will universal health coverage be implemented on the basis of the minimum core concept?[2] If yes, which specific interventions will be included in the minimum core? And what potential will such interventions have to accommodate the adaptation to climate change components? National debate must be encouraged to answer these questions. A view espoused by Forman and colleagues[23] is that strengthening the minimum core "will produce a more feasible and grounded conception of legally prioritized health needs that could assist in advancing health equity, including by providing a framework rooted in legal obligations to guide the formulation of new health development goals, providing a baseline of essential health services to be protected as a matter of right against governmental claims of scarcity and inadequate international assistance, and empowering civil

---

[2] The fact that a nation guarantees a minimum set of standard rights to its people.

society to claim fulfilment of their essential health needs from domestic and global decision-makers".

There is no reason why communities whose poverty is increasing, whose mortality is doubling, whose children are not attending school and whose development is retarded because of repeated floods and droughts linked to climate change should not be compensated for it. The arrangements for such compensation, if not covered by constitutional rights, must be addressed through litigation. Young,[24] when discussing the minimum core of economic and social rights, which includes health, refers to the advocates of the concept, who promote its immediate enforceability and justiciability, including at the constitutional level. Other legal analysts such as Barcellos[25] suggest that "public law litigation can be used to foster public health policies similar to the way in which structural reform litigation and the experimentalism approach between courts and defendants have influenced public policies and achieved institutional reform in schools and prisons".

Yamin[26] in her editorial in the *Health and Human Rights Journal* argues that over the last 20 years, and exponentially in the last decade, there has been an increased enforcement of health and related rights including in Africa and that important demands for health-related entitlements are being framed in terms of legally enforceable claims. The article provides an excellent illustration and case study on access to antiretrovirals by people infected with HIV: "In many ways, the advent of effective anti-retroviral medications (ARVs) in the mid-1990s spawned much of the early health rights litigation. Clear linkages to the right to life, coupled often with issues of discrimination against marginalized groups, and the existence of a clearly defined remedy all contributed to the framing of enforceable legal claims. The existence of important social movements strengthened demands for ARVs in terms of rights, as well as implementation of court decisions, when many political branches of government had previously shown indifference or resistance to providing treatment for people living with HIV/AIDS. Since then, however, health rights litigation has expanded to many other topics, and has begun to have a substantial impact in countries across the world, affecting tens of thousands of individual entitlements to medications and treatments a year in some countries, but also rewriting intellectual property rules, ensuring regulation of laws, causing changes in policies of various kinds, and influencing health priority-setting processes and budgetary allocations".

The health impacts of climate change represent an exciting area to which to expand the right-to-health approaches, including litigation.

One of the community groups most vulnerable to climate change are indigenous people. The African continent has many such groups, for example the pygmies of central Africa and the Maasai of eastern Africa. Social justice compels governments to protect these groups as well as other vulnerable communities. Climate change consequences call for the immediate and effective implementation of the United Nations Declaration on the Rights of Indigenous People.[27] There are specific articles in that declaration that focus on the right to health for such groups as well as the right to manage their natural environments according to their values and traditions. It is clear that protection of indigenous people is interconnected with local environmental governance and safeguarding. But those issues have not yet been sufficiently analysed or acted upon.

Beyond health and human rights, climate change brings into light important governance issues.

These are related to the participation of individuals in the management of public threats and goods. For instance, governments may decide to move entire communities from some 'hazardous' areas to safer locations in the context of climate risk reduction. If the concerned communities are not adequately involved in developing the pertinent policy or in decision-making, such a displacement is likely to fail. Therefore, the approaches used to enhance the participation of communities such as those used in strategic and environmental impact assessments must be extended to the management of the impacts of climate change on health. The objective is to facilitate the full participation of the community and their adherence to the policy options selected and the programmes proposed by the government. Without such engagement, the adaptation or the mitigation programmes will not be effectively implemented.

Political systems themselves are vulnerable to the challenges of climate change. In recent years, a number of countries have witnessed social unrest fuelled by hikes in food prices, which themselves were a consequence of low food production. Climate change has a share in these situations. The unrests upset the stability of the governments of the affected countries and demonstrated the direct impact of climate change on political systems and democracy. Therefore, political issues posed by climate change today are of significantly greater impact than those witnessed during the political transitions in many African countries in the 1990s mentioned above. According to Held and Hervey[28] the "… urgent challenge of climate change poses a critical test for modern democracy and rules based international politics. Democracies need to shift from loose policy commitments to real and binding action. Yet, there are enormous collective action problems in combating climate change".

During the 1990s widespread civil unrests, African people demanded a shift from one party-based political systems to multiparty systems. Many governments at that time conducted large-scale, all-inclusive national policy dialogues, which in many instances led to changes in the national constitution and, consequently, to more viable democracies. Similar or even more powerful political processes are required to address climate change. Although people are not yet demanding these changes, the strong relationship that climate change has with human rights will make these requirements indispensable in the near future. Therefore, governments should act now.

Addressing the impacts of climate change on health as a development opportunity

Addressing public health adaptation to climate change as a development opportunity is concerned with answering the question about how climate change adaptation in public health can positively influence national economies and human development. Job creation and the development of the national expertise could be used to illustrate how climate change adaptation can foster development.

As African countries take on universal health coverage as their new vision and goal in health, they should prioritize low-cost, high-gain interventions. Climate change adaptation can serve as a powerful driver to scale up such interventions, for example in the case of immunization.

Immunization can be considered from the perspective of climate change adaptation. With African governments putting all their efforts to raise immunization coverage to the highest possible levels, it is expected that morbidity and mortality among children will reduce dramatically. The consequences for development from those efforts will be obvious: the overall mortality rates in the countries will decrease sharply, school attendance will rise, more people will achieve higher levels of education and mothers will spend less time looking after ill children and more time in other activities, including income-generating ventures. Household direct expenditure on health, which in Africa is still significant, will decrease and the savings made will be used for other household needs.

What applies to immunization applies also to other climate-sensitive diseases. Scaling up malaria prevention and treatment through existing means, including environmental sanitation and maintenance of such interventions over time, is a way of adapting to climate change. Reducing malaria prevalence in the workforce, for instance, will result in increased productivity.[29]

The other benefits of climate change adaptation for the health sector will be in job creation. Scaling up mitigation and adaptation programmes through the green economy processes will require new and additional expertise in the labour force. For instance, additional health workers will be required to scale up and sustain immunization. Similarly, to manufacture enough clean cooking stoves for nationwide coverage may create hundreds of jobs. Therefore, green job opportunities will emerge in government agencies and enterprises of other stakeholders, including the private sector. As these new jobs are created, new expertise also will be generated. The development of national expertise through training and research will help to consolidate and maintain the gains generated from climate change adaptation health programmes.

Governments need to understand that allocating a part of their national income from the current economic growth and other sources to health adaptation to climate change is certainly one of the best investments they could make. Economic activities are already taking place in Africa driven by the outcomes and decisions from the climate change negotiations under the auspices of UNFCCC. The carbon market and the projects under the UN-REDD (Reducing Emissions from Deforestation and forest Degradation in developing Countries) Programme and those developed to implement the Clean Development Mechanism (CDM) under the UNFCCC instruments are some of the activities already being implemented in many African countries. Unfortunately, the health sector is missing out on these opportunities.

Lambe and colleagues,[30] in a paper entitled 'Can carbon finance transform household energy markets? a review of cook stove projects and programs in Kenya', argue that carbon finance can help build a vibrant market for improved cook stoves by attracting international actors and technologies, helping establish standards for monitoring the manufacture of the stoves, and facilitating follow-up and after-sales support. These programmes and projects offer ample opportunities for health development and for health professionals to work across sectors.

An excellent entry point for health would be in the systematic assessments of the health outcomes of the climate adaptation programmes. Lambe and colleagues[30] recognize that the wood, charcoal and dung used for cooking and heating create serious environmental and health hazards and are responsible for the renewed calls for cleaner and more efficient stoves for people around the world. The need for such solutions is even greater when we consider the desire to reduce deforestation and the cutting of trees, which is the normal practice to satisfy the energy needs of households. One of the expected results will be a substantial reduction in the use of biomass for heating and cooking. This in turn will decrease the amount of particulate matter in the air, improve the air quality and reduce acute respiratory infections.

The health sector needs to understand that it has to more systematically search for opportunities for interlinkages in climate change adaptation processes. Doing so requires stronger ties between health experts and their colleagues in the sectors driving the relevant initiatives such as forestry, agriculture and water. The challenges pertaining to the institution of effective intersectoral actions are known, but they can be overcome through implementing adequate policies and fostering establishment of institutional arrangements.

The global financial architecture for adaptation to and mitigation of climate change is shaping up. The basic principle that guides the various mechanisms being established for developing countries is that the least developed countries and countries with economies in transition, to some extent, need financial compensation for the loss and damage that they are suffering associated with anthropogenic climate change to which their contribution is negligible. As funds are starting to be made available by the Global Green Fund, the African Green Fund and other mechanisms, the ministries of health must prepare and position themselves to attract some of these funds. This can only happen if those ministries are able to develop and articulate their essential key messages on climate change adaptation and communicate them to their counterparts responsible for coordinating and mainstreaming national climate change adaptation and mitigation work or representing them on the international scene. One of such messages could be that climate change is increasing the rate and scope of epidemics (this is true). But when you look at the composition of the African delegations to the UNFCCC Annual Conference of the Parties, you hardly find any health representative. Fortunately, some partners have understood the need to build the capacity of African public health professionals in climate change negotiations and have supported their participation in some of the events. This has remained at an experimental level, though. It is, therefore, up to the ministers of health to understand what their role is and take the necessary action.

Conclusion

African governments have not yet comprehensively assessed the multiple dimensions of climate change or their implications for development in general and public health in particular. They need to carefully study the key messages from climate scientists and take the necessary steps to integrate them into political, social and economic reforms. These reforms will be the condition for viable and effective climate change adaptation and mitigation programmes, especially in the health sector.

The reform process will bring development opportunities with benefits that might outweigh the loss and damage created by climate change. The resources for undertaking the reforms are increasingly becoming available from domestic sources, thanks to economic growth, and the international community. It is now for African leaders to transform the climate change threat into a extraordinary development opportunity. To achieve this it is critical to take 10 important actions:

1. Establish specific climate change and health units within the ministries of health and intersectoral and multidisciplinary public health risk management teams to lead and coordinate national health programmes on adaptation to climate change.

2. Develop and establish national early warning systems with the capacity for undertaking research and developing predictive models on trends in climate change risks and their potential impacts on health.

3. Prepare contingency plans and provide resources and a budget to respond to the acute impacts of extreme weather events in the context of ensuring preparedness for disaster risk management.

4. Establish emergency funds at the level of the ministries of health.

5. Reassess and revise national legislation, including the national constitution, to allow for legal protection of the most vulnerable populations through mechanisms such constitutional rights and litigation.

6. Undertake inclusive national political dialogue to enhance the participation of communities in the adaptation of national political systems to the environmental, social and economic contexts imposed by climate change.

7. Scale up and sustain immunization for the whole population as the best possible climate change adaptation intervention.

8. Develop climate change and health projects that link adaptation to climate change with mitigation of its associated risks, and that create jobs.

9. Systematically include health experts in national delegations to UNFCCC and other international forums to articulate and communicate key messages on health and climate change and to facilitate access to technical and financial resources made available internationally.

10. Develop multisectoral programmes that link health, environment, land and other sectors and that will prioritize the mapping of flood-prone and drought-prone areas, development and implementation of national standards for building and infrastructure construction even for rural settings, identification and preparation of relocation areas, and systematic application of hospital safety criteria.

References

1. UNCTAD. UN list of least developed countries (http://unctad.org/en/pages/aldc/Least%20Developed%20Countries/UN-list-of-Least-Developed-Countries.aspx; accessed 3 March 2015).

2. World Bank. Poverty and Equity Regional Dashboard – sub-Saharan Africa (http://povertydata.worldbank.org/poverty/region/SSA; accessed 3 March 2015).

3. Institute for Health Metrics and Evaluation, Human Development Network, World Bank. 2013. The global burden of disease: generating evidence, guiding policy – sub-Saharan Africa regional edition. Seattle, WA: IHME (http://www.healthdata.org/sites/default/files/files/data_for_download/2013/WorldBank_SubSaharanAfrica/IHME_GBD_WorldBank_SubSaharanAfrica_FullReport.pdf; accessed 3 March 2015).

4. The Lancet. 2009. A commission for climate change. *Lancet* 373(9676):1659–1734.

5. IPCC. 2007. IPCC Fourth Assessment Report: climate change (http://www.ipcc.ch/publications_and_data/ar

4/syr/en/mains1.html; accessed 26 February 2015).

6. UNFCCC. Climate change – Term Definition (http://unfccc.int/files/documentation/text/html/; accessed 26 February 2015).

7. United States Environmental Protection Agency. Climate change: basic information (http://www.epa.gov/climatechange/basics/; accessed 26 February 2015).

8. IIPCC. 2013. Climate change: the Physical Science Basis Working Group I contribution to the Fifth Assessment Report of the Intergovernmental Panel on Climate Change (http://www.ipcc.ch/pdf/assessment-report/ar5/wg1/WG1AR5_Frontmatter_FINAL.pdf; accessed on 26 February 2015).

9. Held D and Hervey AF. 2009. Democracy, climate change and global governance: democratic agency and the policy menu ahead. Policy Network (www.policy-network.net; accessed 22 March 2015).

10. Global Framework for Climate Services (http://www.gfcs-climate.org; accessed on 19 March 2015).

11. Thomson MC, Mason S, Platzer B, Mihretie A, Omumbo J, Mantilla G, Ceccato P, Jancloes M and Connor S. 2014. Climate and Health in Africa. Earth Perspectices,1:17.

12.   Alonso D, Bouma MJ, Pascual M. 2011. Epidemic malaria and warmer temperatures in recent decades in an east African highlands. *Proc Biol Sci.* 278(1712): 1661–1669.

13. Byass P. 2009. Climate change and population health in Africa: where are the scientists? Global Health Action (http://www.globalhealthactionnet/index.php/gha/article/view/2065/2504; accessed 26 February 2015).

14. WHO. 2009. Global health risks: mortality and burden of disease attributable to selected major risks. World Health Organization, Geneva.

15. WHO. 2012. *Atlas of health and climate.* World Health Organization, Geneva.

16. Luber G, Knowlton K, Balbus J, Frumkin H, Hayden M, Hess J, McGeehin M, Sheats N, Backer L, Beard CB, Ebi KL, Maibach E, Ostfeld RS, Wiedinmyer C, Zielinski-Gutiérrez E and Ziska L. 2014. Human health climate change impacts in the United States: In: Melillo JM, Richmond TTC, Yohe GW, eds, *The third national climate assessment.* U.S. Global Change Research Program. p 220–256. doi:10.7930/J0PN93H5.

17. Manga L, Bagayoko M, Meredith T, Neira M. 2013. Overview of health considerations

within national adaptation programmes of action for climate change in least developed countries and small island states. *African Health Monitor*, March 2013.

18. WHO. 2012. Adaptation to climate change in Africa: plan of action for the health sector, 2012–2016. World Health Organization, Regional Office for Africa, Brazzaville.

19. The Disaster and Emergency Management Presidency of Turkey http://en.wikipedia.org/wiki/Disaster_and_E mergency_Management_Presidency; accessed 1 March 2015).

20. The Government of Mexico and the WorldBank. 2012. Improving the assessment of disaster risks to strengthen financial resilience. In: *Disaster risk management in Mexico: from response to risk transfer.* The World Bank, Washington, DC.

21. The World Bank. 2012. An efficient strategy to prevent and manage disaster risks in Mexico (http://www.worldbank.org/en/news/feature/2 012/11/20/strategy-to-prevent-and-manage-disaster-risks-Mexico; accessed 1 March 2015).

22. Mutangadura G, Gauci A, Armah B, Woldemariam E, Ayalew D, Egu B. 2007. Health inequities in selected African countries: review of evidence and policy implications (http://www.afdb.org/fileadmin/uploads/afdb/Documents/Knowledge/Conference_2007_an glais_21-part-V-1.pdf; accessed 22 March 2015).

23. Forman L, Ooms G, Chapman A, Friedman E, Waris A, Lamprea E, Mulumba M. 2013. What could a strengthened right to health bring to the post-2015 health development agenda? – interrogating the role of the minimum core concept in advancing essential global health needs. *International Health and Human Rights* 13(48) (http://www.biomedcentral.com/1472-698X/13/48. Accessed on 12 June 2015)

24. Young KG. 2008. The minimum core of economic and social rights: a concept in search of content. *Yale Journal of International Law* 33(113), 113-175.

25. Barcellos AP. 2014. Sanitation rights, public law litigation, and inequality: a case study from Brazil. *Health and Human Rights Journal* 16(2). http://www.hhrjournal.org/2014/09/23/sanitation-rights-public-law-litigation-and-inequality-a-case-study-from-brazil/(accessed on 12 June 2015).

26. Yamin AE. 2014. Promoting equity in health: what role for courts? *Health and Human Rights Journal*, 16(2). Editorial.

27. UN. United Nations Declaration on the Rights of Indigeneous Peoples. (http://www.un.org/esa/socdev/unpfii/documents/DRIPS_en.pdf; accessed 22 March 2015).

28. Held D, Hervey AF. 2009. Democracy, climate change and global governance: democratic agency and the policy menu ahead. Policy Network (www.policy-network.net; accessed 22 March 2015).

29. Dillon A, Friedman J, Serneels P. 2014. Experimental evidence from malaria testing and treatment among Nigerian sugarcane cutters. The World Bank Group. WPS7120. Washington DC.

30. Lambe F, Jürisoo M, Lee C, Johnson O. 2015. Can carbon finance transform household energy markets? A review of cookstove projects and programs in Kenya.

Energy Research and Social Sciences 5:55–66.